A Month of Happiness with Ms. Mollie

A Month of Happiness with Ms. Mollie

Healthy Recipes for 31
Days of Daily Living

Mollie Ann Holt

For Speaking Engagements, Radio and Television Interviews:
Contact
Ms Mollie Ann Holt
310-321-2390
mollieannholt@gmail.com

ISBN:	Hardcover	978-1-9845-3225-1
	Softcover	978-1-9845-3139-1
	eBook	978-1-9845-3138-4

Print information available on the last page.

Rev. date: 06/15/2018

To order additional copies of this book, contact:
Xlibris
1-888-795-4274
www.Xlibris.com
Orders@Xlibris.com
780038

Contents

This Book is dedicated to the memory of my both my grandparents, and my belated, Sport and Entertainment Attorney, James Nasos Mancuso, ESQ in California who taught me how to pursue my dreams until the end. Gunnstaks Law Office in Plano, Texas over my Talent Agency called, Mollie Global Inc. Talent Agency who believes in my talents and taught me how to stay focused on my goals. My sweet friend, my confidant, prayer warrior, mentor Grace R. Milligan, and great friend, Sheena Ayers in Houston, Texas. Most of all, my heavenly father who gave me my unique, talents and only father in the face of adversity.

Acknowledgments

I wish to thank my creator who gave me my unique, talents.

To my confidant, and God mother in Texas.

To all of my talent in my agency I encouraged to be more than they are today.

To my two entertainment attorneys in Texas and California.

To Wolf Entertainment Production and the CHD Community. You are very special people who needs more research on CHD at birth.

Authors Notes

This book is intended for entertainment purposes only!

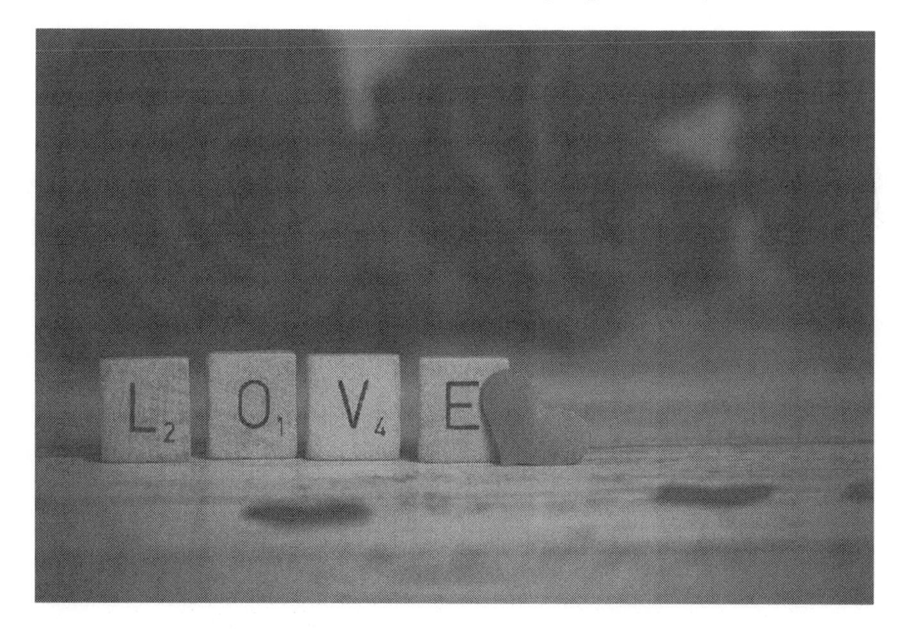

Chapter 1

HEALTHY RECIPES FOR DAILY LIVING

Healthy recipe
How to Pamper Yourself
Quote from Ms. Mollie Ann Holt

Day- 1: Recipe: Festive Fruit, Nut, & Chocolate Chip Balls Rolled in Coconut

Ingredients

3/4 cup sugar
1/2 cup dried cranberries
1/2 cup pitted and snipped dates
2 large eggs, beaten
1/3 cup chopped pistachios, preferably unsalted
1/3 cup chopped walnuts
1/3 cup chopped pecans
1 teaspoon rum extract
3/4 cup shredded coconut

Preparation

Mix all ingredients together and make balls.

2. Something just for you:

Take a lavender bath to calm your nerves at night. Always add Epson salt to get rid of all of the people you need to peel away. This keeps you refreshed. Just ask me! It is the minerals.

Secret Tip

Rolling them in shredded coconut gives them their festive look.

3. Quote for the day:

A spoonful of kisses a day and a dash of love go a long way.

Day 2 – Recipe "Egg & Salmon Sandwich with half an orange"

Ingredients

1/2 teaspoon extra-virgin olive oil
1 tablespoon finely chopped red onion
2 large egg whites, beaten
Pinch of salt
1/2 teaspoon capers, rinsed and chopped (optional)
1 ounce smoked salmon
1 slice tomato
1 whole-wheat English muffin, split and toasted

Preparation

Toast the English muffin, place, egg whites, tomato slices, capers, salmon, and chopped onions. Then, squeeze a little lemon for flavor.

2. Something just for you:

Put a cucumber peel on your face to exfoliate the days dust. Then, soak in a mineral bath to rid yourself of all the people that sucked you dry of life! Just ask me! It is the minerals that do the job! Got to love that!

Secret tip

Add squeezed lemon for a zesty flavor on the salmon before you close the sandwich.

3. Quote for the day:

"When you get P.A.I.N. in your life, it only means: Positive Attitude In Negative Situations.

Day 3 – Recipe "Luscious Rack of Lamb with Baked Zucchini Squash"

Ingredients

Minced garlic
Fresh rosemary
Dijon mustard
Sea salt
Cracked pepper
Egg Yokes
1 medium zucchini squash
Butter
lemon
Baking sheet

Preparation

Preheat oven to 450° and use a gas or charcoal grill for the lamb.

Directions:

First, smother eggs yokes and Dijon mustard all over the rack of lamb. Let it stand for 1 hour on a baking sheet. Then, bake in the oven for 15 minutes. Place fresh rosemary on top. Then, a touch of sea salt, and little cracked pepper. Minced garlic goes on top. Last, cut the zucchini in half, and brush some butter, and lemon on top. Serve.

Secret tip

The Dijon mustard will give it a kick.

2. Something just for you:

Get a cylinder foam roller that you can roll out the knots in your body. Use it daily! It releases so much tension during a long day.

3. Quote of the day:

Strength involves body, mind, and spirit through.

Day 4: Recipe: "Marinated Olives & Feta with a Flatbread"

Ingredients

1 cup sliced pitted olives, such as Kalamata or mixed Greek
1/2 cup diced feta cheese, preferably reduced-fat
2 tablespoons extra-virgin olive oil
Zest and juice of 1 lemon
2 cloves garlic, sliced
1 teaspoon chopped fresh rosemary
Pinch of crushed red pepper
Freshly ground pepper to taste
Hot pickled sliced jalapenos (as many as you want)

Secret tip

Cover and refrigerate up to a day

Combine olives, feta, oil, lemon zest and juice, garlic, rosemary, crushed red pepper and black pepper in a medium bowl.

2. Something just for you:

Sit in a Jacuzzi with bubbles, outside in the moonlight. Or, do a bubble bath and just soak. Then, take melatonin and sleep sound.

Quote of the day:

"Forgiveness frees your soul".

Day 5 - Recipe: "Fabulous Filet Mignon with Candy Carrots"

Ingredients

4 oz., 1 & half inch filet mignon, all natural, prime, angus steak
Black pepper
1 stick Real organic butter
Sea salt
Carrots
1 cup of Brown Sugar
Feta cheese
French crispy Onions
Olive oil
Scallions
Medium sauce pan

Preparation

Use a gas grill at 450 degrees and get it to high heat. Cook both sides for 7 minutes each and no more than 15 minutes.

Take the filet migon, and place a little sea salt on top. Just a little bit.

Cut carrots and place in the sauce pan with brown sugar, and butter and bring to a boil until it caramelizes.

Take the scallions and put in a sauce pan with a teaspoon of butter and sauté for ten minutes.

After the steak is ready, top with crumbled, feta cheese, drizzle olive oil, and last the French, crispy, onions.

Secret Tip

Gas grill is the best and a charcoal grill to make it a smoked flavor. I prefer charcoal since I like seasonings. Also, on the carrots sprinkle some cinnamon.

Something just for you:

Go and get a manicure and pedicure. Do a massage at the same time on your shoulders.

Quote of the day:

> "Don't let the tumbleweeds of life suck you into the ground".

Day 6 – Recipe "Shrimp Tacos with Blueberry-Avocado Salsa"

Ingredients

1 teaspoon garlic powder
¼ teaspoon of cumin
¼ teaspoon of chili powder
¼ teaspoon of paprika
1 teaspoon of fresh lime juice
5oz of shrimp
1 teaspoon of olive oil
¼ chopped avocado
¼ chopped blueberries
1 tablespoon chopped fresh cilantro
1 teaspoon of fresh lime juice
Dash of salt and pepper
2 corn tortillas
1 tablespoon of Greek nonfat plain yogurt

Preparation

In a bowl, combine garlic, cumin, chili powder, paprika, fresh lime, toss in shrimp that is deveined and peeled, and marinate shrimp, add the olive oil. Cook for ten minutes. In a bowl, combine the blueberries, avocado, cilantro, lime juice, salt, and pepper. Take the two corn tortillas and spread the Greek yogurt.

Secret Tip

Add crushed jalapenos to the shrimp. It adds a kick. Plus these are a great form of antioxidants.

Something just for you:

Take a walk in the park for three, and take your favorite music and get lost in the words.

Quote of the day:

"Strength involves fitness of body, mind, and spirit".

Day 7 – Recipe: "Apple Fennel Salad with Blue Cheese"

Ingredients:

1/4 cup extra-virgin olive oil
2 tablespoons cider vinegar
1/4 teaspoon salt
1/4 teaspoon freshly ground pepper
1 large crisp, sweet apple, such as Honey crisp or Ambrosia, thinly sliced
1 medium fennel bulb, quartered and thinly sliced, fronds reserved
6 cups torn butter head lettuce
1/3 cup crumbled blue cheese

Preparation

Whisk oil, vinegar, salt and pepper in a large bowl. Add apple and fennel and toss to coat. Chop 1/4 cup of the fennel fronds and add to the bowl along with lettuce and blue cheese; gently toss.

Secret tip

Used green apples for flavor.

Something just for you:

Write in a journal, your dreams and desires. Then, don't forget to lock it up in a safe place so no finds it. It is between you and our heavenly father.

Quote of the day:

> "Illustrate the power of quiet strength in resisting oppression and injustice.

Day 8 – Recipe "Pear Slices with Almond Butter"

Ingredients

1 tablespoon of almond butter
¼ teaspoon of powdered ginger
½ medium pear sliced

Preparation

Combine almond butter and powdered ginger, and spread it on the pear slices.

Secret tip

Drizzle some honey. Home grown honey helps cure allergies.

2. Something just for you:

Find a movie and lose yourself. What I mean is get into someone else's world.

3. Quote of the day:

> "Until I die, my life does not have a finish line".

Day 9 – Recipe "Guilt Free Italian, Lightened Up Chicken Parmesan"

Ingredients

4 boneless chicken breasts (4 oz.)
Dash of Garlic salt
Canola Oil cooking spray
¼ cup of whole wheat flour
1 egg & 1 egg white
4 cups of cornflakes finely crushed
1 teaspoon Italian seasoning
1 cup of homemade or jarred marinara with lots of minced garlic
4 tablespoon of grated parmesan
1 cup of shredded provolone cheese

Preparation

Heat oven to 375 degrees. Pound chicken between two sheets of plastic wrap until ¼ inch thick. Unwrap and season with garlic salt. Coat cooking sheet with canola oil. In a bowl place flour. In second bowl place egg and egg white beaten. In a third bowl, combine corn flakes and Italian seasoning. Coat chicken with all the above. Place chicken on sheet and bake for 8 minutes. Top chicken with ¼ cup of marinara and 1 tablespoon of grated cheese, and bake for 5 minutes.

Secret tip

Add extra olive oil for flavor.

2. Something just for you:

Have a glass of your favorite wine and read some old love stories.

3. Quote of the day:

> "In a changing world, an open mind is your strongest ally".

Day 10 – Recipe "French Toast with Honey and Powdered Sugar"

Ingredients

Two slices of wheat bread
Two egg whites
Two tablespoons of vanilla almond milk
¼ teaspoon of cinnamon
1 tablespoon of honey
1 tablespoon of olive oil
pepper
1 tablespoon of real unsalted butter

Preparation

Whip the egg whites, vanilla almond milk, mix in the cinnamon, and pepper. Then, soak bread in the egg mixture. Place in a skillet and put butter in the pan. Place on medium heat. Cook until it is the way you like it.

Secret tip

The wheat flour processes much better in the body due to the grains.

2. Something just for you:

Curl up in your favorite chair, no dressing up, be casual, and have "tea time" on the phone with a new friend.

3. Quote of the day:

> "Often strength lies in restraint, in not responding".

Day 11 – Recipe "Mollie's Fitness Breakfast"

Ingredients

4oz lean ground round red or turkey meat
8oz of oatmeal, grits, malto meal, cream of rice or wheat
1 scoop of protein in 8oz or 12oz of water
1 multivitamin & 1000mg of vitamin C
½ grapefruit

Preparation

Grill the meat in a skillet with olive oil, fresh lemon, and pepper. Add honey to your oatmeal, grits, etc.

Secret tip

Drink water by itself doing cardio with a fat burner. You burn more bad fat in the morning. I am a physical and pageant trainer, a U.S. pageant judge and Ms. Fitness qualifier, judge. Take caution at first and seek advice of a doctor consuming any supplements. They all have side effects.

2. Something just for you:

Go for a walk in a park with a plastic sweat suit from head to toe and a rubber waist band. Make certain you put your favorite music that jack up the walk a notch. I can refer you!

3. Quote for the day:

> "When you take a step to a better body, your heavenly father takes a step to help achieve it".

Day 12 – Recipe "M.A.H. Creations Cookies"

Ingredients

2 and 1/4 cups of wheat flour
1 teaspoon of baking soda
1 teaspoon of salt
1 teaspoon of baking powder
¾ cup of sugar in the raw and brown sugar
1 cup of semi-sweet chocolate chips
1 tablespoons of almond
1 cup of maraschino cherries chopped
2 eggs, organic, brown, and uncaged
2 stick of real organic butter
2 tablespoon of real vanilla
1 cup chopped walnuts nuts
Add tablespoon of rum

Preparation

Heat oven to 350 degrees. Then, mix flour mixture in one bowl. Then, mix eggs, almond, rum, butter, in another in another bowl. Combine both. Then, add the cherries, chocolate chips, and walnuts last. Drop by tablespoon on a cookie sheet. Grease the cookie sheet with Bakers spray.

Secret tip

Add real rum to the mix to make it divine.

2. Something just for you:

Go to Las Vegas and sing at a Karaoke place. Then, have the entire place give you a standing ovation for a show. Ask me! I did it with a darling friend! It is invigorating.

3. Quote for the day:

> "Everyone comes with baggage. Find someone who loves you enough to unpack the baggage and do the same for them".

Day 13 – Recipe "Fresh Herb Linguine"

1 pound fresh or frozen peeled, deveined medium shrimp
6 ounces packaged dried linguini or spaghetti
1/4 cup grated Parmesan cheese
4 cloves garlic, minced
2 tablespoons extra-virgin olive oil
1 1/2 teaspoons snipped fresh rosemary
1/2 teaspoon salt
1/2 teaspoon coarsely ground black pepper
Rosemary sprigs (optional)

Preparation

Thaw shrimp, if frozen. Rinse shrimp and set aside. Cook pasta according to package directions, omitting any salt and fat. Add the shrimp the last 3 minutes of cooking. Drain well and place in a large pasta bowl. Add 2 tablespoons of the cheese, the garlic, olive oil, snipped rosemary, salt and black pepper and toss until well coated. Sprinkle evenly with the 2 tablespoons remaining cheese and garnish with rosemary sprigs, if desired. Makes 4 servings (1 cup each)

Secret tip

Add lots of garlic, and olive oil.

2. Something just for you:

Go to a secret shop where you can only buy a one of a kind item. Then, keep your mouth shut.

3. Quote for the day

"Is your glass half full, or is half empty"?

Day 14 – Recipe "Succulent, Poached, Eggs with Roma Stewed Tomatoes and Asparagus"

Ingredients

Two large, white eggs
Fresh Roma tomatoes
Fresh garlic cloves
Ground black pepper
Purple onions
Asparagus
Basil
Grated Parmesan
Lemon
Parmesan cheese
White vinegar
Sea salt
2 quart sauce pan
Inch high water

Directions

Take two large, white, eggs and make certain the eggs are really cold.

Get a two quart sauce pan, heat water to boiling stage for fifteen minutes

Take out of boiling water into a large bowl filled with ice and refrigerate for 8 hours. Reheat in warm water just before serving.

Place a teaspoon of salt, and two teaspoons of vinegar in the boiling water.

Use a rounded spatula to pick up the poached egg.

Chop a purple onion and sauté in the skillet with fresh lime.

Preparation

After you take out the poached eggs, put a touch of sea salt, and sautéed onions and top. Place the fresh asparagus on top of the poached eggs. Then, sprinkle parmesan on top of the stewed cold tomatoes on the side. Squeeze fresh lemon on top of the tomatoes.

Secret tip

Add garlic cloves in the boiling water for flavor and taste.

2. **Something just for you**:

Go challenge your exercise routine. Make some changes like higher levels on a cardio equipment.

3. Quote for the day:

"Be Fearless".

Day 16 – Recipe "Detox Water"

Ingredients

2 lemons
½ cucumber
10 to 12 mint leaves
4 quarts of water

Preparation

Brew overnight. Then, drink all day. This is for keeping a flat stomach.

Secret tip

Do a colon cleanse first. Use Mega Cleanse every six months.

2. Something Just for You:

Do an obstacle course that challenges your core.

3. Quote for the day:

"Step up the pace in your life.

Day 17 – Recipe "Dark & White Chocolate Cranberry Clusters"

Ingredients

2 bags 8 ounces of fresh cranberries
1 bag of 8 ounce white chocolate morsels
1 bag of 8 ounce dark chocolate morsels

Preparation

Heat on the stove the chocolates until melted. Then, mix in the cranberries. Afterwards, take a tablespoon and scoop out enough on drop on a piece of wax paper. Let cool until solid. Then, you have a beautiful, perfect, chocolate, cranberry cluster.

Secret Tip

You must put in fresh vanilla for taste. Do not put imitation. You can use the bakers blocks chocolate squares for proper molding.

2. Pamper yourself, "Do soul surgery on your soul". That means break down everything in your life that needs forgiveness. Then, go to the people you need to ask forgiveness. What this does is restores your soul. As a result, this is called "soul surgery".

3. Quote for the day,

"Soak yourself in other languages".

Day 18 – Recipe “Green Goddess and Vegetable Sticks”

Ingredients

Celery sticks
Baby Carrots
Green Goddess Dressing
Small Dixie cups

Preparation

Take the Dixie cups and place six sticks in the cup, and place a ¼ of Green Goddess dressing in the bottom.

Secret tip

Place three cherry tomatoes for color and flavor and great for holiday colors.

2. Something just for you:

“Go buy something that makes you feel and look priceless”.

3. Quote for the day:

> “Dream big with high desirable expectations like you never have dreamed before”. Remember, winners never quit.

Day 19 – Recipe “Pear Salad with Grilled Shrimp”

Ingredients

10 ounces spring mix salad
½ cup pecans, chopped
½ cup of dried cranberries
1/4 cup feta cheese, crumbled

Pear, cored, and sliced with skin
1/3 cup of Creamy Balsamic with Herbs dressing
8 ounces of shrimp

Preparation

In a bowl, slice up the pears, add pecans, feta cheese, and mix in dressing. Then, place the shrimp on top.

Secret tip

Add the dried cranberries for flavor.

2. Something just for you:

"Surround yourself around people who appreciate your presence".

3. Quote for the day:

"Never, ever, quit your dreams".

Day 20 – Recipe – "Christmas Chocolate S'mores with Maraschino Cherries"

Ingredients

Nabisco honey graham crackers
1 bag of large marsh mellows
1 bag of Hershey's chocolate bars
Jar of maraschino red and green cherries
Mint extract

Preparation

Preheat your over to 350 degrees. Take a graham cracker and break into half. Then, take a large marsh mellow open it and stick the red or green cherries into the marsh mellow, and add a tiny square of chocolate on each side and put on a non-stick cookie sheet and bake at 8 minutes at 350 degrees. Make certain you do not overcook.

Secret tip

Place a little drop of mint for taste.

2. Something just for you:

Declutter your life by cleaning out things you do not need collecting dust in your home or office. Then, reorganize. I cannot understand pack rats. Remember, we do not die with possessions.

3. Quote for the day:

> "Strengthen your heart muscles by lifting someone else's spirits".

Day 21 – Recipe: "Chocolate Dipped, Banana & Strawberry Skewer"

Ingredients

California strawberries
Ripe bananas
White and dark baking squares
Skewer sticks
4 tablespoons of chocolate Godiva liquor

Preparation

Heat stove to medium, in two different medium sauce pots, heat up the white and dark baking squares, place 4 tablespoons of chocolate Godiva liquor and stir until melted. Make certain you do not over heat the chocolate. Take large strawberries and cut up two inch bananas and slide on skewers. Dip each one in different chocolate by using a tablespoon. Drizzle white choc on strawberries, and dark chocolate on bananas.

Secret tip

The last thing you want to do is sprinkle powdered sugar on the top of the finished skewer for a pretty effect and sweet finish. These are my favorite at Christmas time.

2. Something just for you:

"Give yourself some private time each day to reflect on accomplishments."

3. Quote for the day:

> "Send out love to all the people who do not know how to love you back, and then let it go".

Day 22 – Recipe "Croissant Italian Sausage Wraps"

Ingredients

1 can of Pillsbury croissants
1 small roll of mild or spicy Italian sausage
4 ounces of black olives chopped
Minced garlic
4 ounces of pepperchinis

Preparation

Preheat your over per the croissants instructions. Then, on the stove, sauté the uncooked Italian sausage, chopped olives, minced garlic, and the pepperchinis until browned. Then, open the croissants and take a tablespoon and fold it and place on a non-stick cooking sheet and bake for 8 to 10 minutes. Make certain the croissant is cooked all the way through so it is not doughy.

Secret tip

The pepperchinis give it a kick and flavor. I love these Italian hot peppers. They are a party in my mouth. My first crush was an Italian sausage. I was 17 years old and he was 21. My daddy said, no! I said, why? I love him! He said, no you're too young. That Italian sausage taught me about wine and how to make gravy.

2. **Something just for you**:

"Cleanse your mind, body, and soul purging daily".

3. Quote for the day:

"Have a purpose in life and profit from it"!

Day 23 – Recipe "Sunset Dip"

Ingredients

One 8 ounce cream cheese softened
4 ounces shredded Mexican mixed cheddar cheese
1 cup of pace picante hot sauce
1 teaspoon of fresh minced garlic
1 tablespoon of olive oil

Preparation

Take a round glass bowl or decorate round glass bowl and spread the cream cheese, mixed with minced garlic, and a tablespoon of olive oil. Then, take cheddar cheese and spread it around showing a little of the white edge of the cream cheese, then put in the middle the Pace Picante hot sauce. You should then have a beautiful picture of a sunset. Heat in the microwave to melt the cheddar so you look like it has sun rays.

Secret tip

For more a healthier chip use wheat tortilla chips.

2. Something just for yourself:

"Try something you have never done before".

3. Quote for the day:

"Challenge yourself to conquer your dreams".

Day 24 – Recipe "Sweet & Sassy Meatballs"

Ingredients

1 box of stuffing chicken and herbs
2 pounds of ground beef
2 eggs
Minced garlic
4 tablespoons of real butter
One 16 ounce can of jellied cranberry sauce
One 8 ounce can of crushed pineapple
One 18 ounce, jar of barbeque sauce
Olive oil

Preparation

Heat skillet on the stove add the butter. Mix stuffing mixture, ground beef, eggs, garlic, and olive oil together and make two inch balls. Place in the skillet and cook until browned and meat is cooked. Afterwards, take the jellied cranberry sauce, crushed pineapples, and barbeque sauce and set aside. Put meatballs on low heat and put this sassy sauce in the meatballs. Should make about two dozen meatballs.

Secret tip

Use organic brown eggs. Also, put a little touch of Tabasco sauce in the sauce for a hot kick.

2. Something just for yourself: "Buy yourself your favorite flowers, and send them to yourself with a card that says "you're an awesome human being".

3. Quote for the day:

"Dream it, believe it, and achieve it".

Day 25 – Recipe: "Chicken Chili with Cannellini Beans"

3 cups tortilla chips
1 pound skinless, boneless chicken breasts or thighs, cut in bite-size pieces
2 teaspoons olive oil
Two, 19 ounce, can of cannellini beans, rinsed, and drained
8 ounces shredded Monterey Jack cheese with jalapeno peppers (1-1/2 cups)
One 4 1/2 ounce can diced green chilies
One 18 ounce can reduced sodium chicken broth
½ cup of fresh cilantro

Preparation

Place all the above in a stew pot big enough for 4 to 5 quarts. Add all ingredients together, and then place grated cheddar and crushed. Tortilla, lime, wheat chips on top of the chili.

Secret tip

Mix in ½ cup of fresh cilantro. Also, the lime, wheat, tortilla chips, are best on top. If you prefer a little chopped jalapenos on top, go ahead in dive into some sin.

2. Something just for yourself: "Make a 5 course dinner for yourself, with candles, your favorite beverage, and some of your favorite music".

3. Quote for the day:

"Live like it is your birthday everyday". I do! Just ask my friend, Cheri.

Day 26 – Recipe "Ms. Mollie's Pimento Cheese with Kick"

Ingredients

2/3 cup small, sliced, pimiento, green olives (from 10-ounce jar)
16 small green olives with pimentos
2 cups finely, shredded Cheddar cheese (4 ounces)
1/4 cup mayonnaise with olive oil
1 low fat package cream cheese, softened (3 ounces)
¼ cup of chives
Dash ground red pepper (cayenne)
16 slices cocktail rye bread
¼ chopped hot or mild jalapenos

Preparation

In a bowl mix all of the wet and dry ingredients above. Then, take the small rye square breads and put on two tablespoons of pimento spread. Then, take a colored, plastic, toothpick and take a small olive and stick it onto the top of the bread. Then, sprinkle a touch of cayenne pepper on top for color. You have a holiday effect.

Secret tip

Add the hot jalapeños for flavor. These are antioxidants and will cleanse out your system. Just ask me and we can talk about it.

2. Something just for yourself:

"Start with a journal, then write a book about your life, and make a movie out of it".

3. Quote for the day:

"Pray for the impossible to occur, and then act on the impossible".

Day 27 – Recipe "Strawberries Delight Dessert"

Ingredients

8 ounces of light sour cream
½ cup of brown sugar
¼ cup of powdered sugar
California large strawberries

Preparation

You must have two small, cute dipping bowls for sour cream and brown sugar. Take the strawberry, dip it into the sour cream first, then the brown sugar, and sprinkle the powdered sugar on top to pull all the flavors together.

Secret tip

Serve with quiche Lorraine with a sweet crust. The powder sugar is what makes the crust sweet.

2. Something just for you:

"Get a new haircut, change the color when you feel you need change in your life, and then change your environment".

3. Quote for the day:

"When you fail to plan, you plan to fail".

Day 28 – Recipe "Fruity, Fantastic, Oatmeal"

Ingredients

One 8 ounce bag of plain instant oatmeal ready for microwave
¼ cup of sliced almonds

¼ cup of dried cranberries
1/4 cup of vanilla almond milk (add more if needed)

Preparation

Put in microwave to cook the oatmeal, and vanilla almond milk. Then, add in the almonds, and the cranberries.

Secret tip

Add a touch of real vanilla in the oatmeal and a dash of cinnamon on top.

2. Something just for you:

"Get a facial, massage, pedicure, and manicure at your favorite salon". Make certain, you dip your hands in hot wax. It makes your hands feel like silk. I love it!

3. Quote for the day:

"Aging is not lost youth, but a new stage".

Day 29 – Recipe "Sweet Pie Crust"

Ingredients

2 cups of wheat flour
¼ teaspoon of salt
½ teaspoon of granulated sugar
¼ powdered sugar
1 cup of vegetable shortening
½ cup of ice water

Preparation

For the crust: In a mixing bowl, combine the flour, salt and sugar. Add the shortening and work it through with your hands until the mixture resembles coarse crumbs. Add the water, 1 tablespoon at a time, and work it in with your hands until you have a smooth ball of dough. Wrap the dough in plastic and refrigerate for at least 30 minutes. Remove the dough from the refrigerator and place it on a lightly floured surface. This recipe makes two pie crusts.

Take your hands rub the wheat flour in your hands so it does not stick to your hands. Then, get your non-stick, round pie shells and get the dough and press with your hands.

Secret tip

The sweetness of the crust is due to the powdered sugar. My grandma taught me this with her all of her pies. I added the wheat crust since it processes better with the metabolism.

2. Something just for you:

Be in silence all day long. That means shut the world out for one solid day. Your voice needs a rest to recharge. Have a chai tea to enhance your voice.

3. Quote for the day:

"Life is as beautiful as you make it".

Day 30 – Recipe "Ms. Mollie's Quiche Lorraine"

Ingredients

Filing for Quiche

8 slices apple wood, bacon, crisply cooked, crumbled (1/2 cup)
1 cup shredded Swiss and Cheddar cheese (4 oz.)
1/3 cup finely chopped onion

4 large, brown, organic, uncaged, eggs
2 cups half-and-half
1/4 teaspoon sea salt
1/4 teaspoon pepper
1/8 teaspoon ground red pepper (cayenne)
Pie shell for "Sweet Pie Crust"
2 cups of wheat flour
¼ teaspoon of salt
½ teaspoon of granulated sugar
¼ powdered sugar
1 cup of vegetable shortening
½ cup of ice water

Preparation – Pie Crust

Heat oven at 425 and bake crust for 9 minutes.

For the crust: In a mixing bowl, combine the flour, salt and sugar. Add the shortening and work it through with your hands until the mixture resembles coarse crumbs. Add the water, 1 tablespoon at a time, and work it in with your hands until you have a smooth ball of dough. Wrap the dough in plastic and refrigerate for at least 30 minutes. Remove the dough from the refrigerator and place it on a lightly floured surface. This recipe makes two pie crusts.

Take your hands rub the wheat flour in your hands so it does not stick to your hands. Then, get your non-stick, round pie shells and get the dough and press with your hands.

Preparation – Filling

Heat the oven 325 and bake for 45 to 50 minutes. Mix the eggs in a separate bowl, sea salt, cayenne pepper, half and half, and real vanilla. Place the crumbled apple wood, bacon in the bottom first. Add the onions next. The egg mixture goes last.

Secret tip

Sauté the onions in real organic butter. Also, add fresh minced garlic to the onions.

2. Something just for you:

"Say thank you for everything you got that day". That means say thank you for the money that paid for all the things you have received that day! At the end of the day the money is not yours. Remember, we do not die with money or material possessions.

3. Quote for the day:

"Count your blessings every day, and list them".

Day 31 – Recipe "Chocolate, Cherry & Carmel, Dipped Apples"

Ingredients

1 package of dark baking blocks that look like ice cubes
1 jar of maraschino cherries
I bag of caramels
1 bag of gala apples
Bag of plastic skewer sticks

Preparation

Heat on the stove in separate pots the chocolate and caramel. Get plastic stick and puncture a hole in the top of the apple. Dip it into the chocolate and drizzle the caramel all around the apple with a teaspoon. Chop up the cherries and roll the apple before all wet stuff dries. I promise the chocolate will dry fast.

Secret tip

Sprinkle powdered sugar on top to make it festive.

2. Something just for you:

“Say the words “I love you to yourself” and be proud of your accomplishments. Most people could care less about your accomplishments, unless they know your character, heart, and soul”.

3. Quote for the day:

> “Dream bigger then you have ever imagined, then do the dream as big as you can without ceasing”.

Chapter 2

RECIPE FOR GREAT INGREDIENTS REGARDING YOUR OWN RELATIONSHIP (PERSONAL OR PROFESSIONAL)

Recipe for Great Ingredients Regarding Your Own Relationships (personal or professional)

Preheat that friendship in the beginning at 250 degrees and then bake forever at five hundred degrees. It is important to make certain of all your important ingredients before you start baking. Afterwards, place in the oven and watch things rise.

Special Note: If it boils over, you either hit a home run or you're out forever sitting out on the side lines in life. If it boils over really bad, plead the 5th and I am sorry to say you will have to chapter 13 that friendship. Then, you figure out you redo the recipe and change up your ingredients. Specific ingredients, like communication or love that were stale in the beginning you realize it was never meant to be stirred up in the first place. Mixing any of the ingredients will probably explode in front of your face and will end up in a family attorney. If you need some, I can assist. On the other hand, a recipe filled with quality ingredients baked in the beginning requires a special ingredient called attention. This vital ingredient called attention provides an explosive, successful, healthy, and satisfying recipe for a lasting friendship.

Furthermore, add the vital ingredient attention in your personal and professional friendships at all times.

Here are some vital ingredients to use sparingly.

Ingredients:

Add affection
Add romance
Add attention
Add prayer time together
Add communication
Add motivation
Add tender loving care
Add kisses
Add grace
Add hugs
Add trust

Add unconditional love
Add in faith
Add truth serum (wine or whatever your poison)
Add Epson salt
Add whispers
Add logic
Add your soul
Add your heart
Add commitment
Add compromise
Add a prenuptial agreement (Our creator does not want our material possessions, he wants our souls.)
Add a family attorney with a sense of humor
Add healthy food
Add respect
Add sincerity
Add humor
Add water
Add sex
Add superglue

First, you must start by adding an unconditional friend that you simmer for whatever time you feel is just right for a special baking recipe. Then, if you feel want to kick it up a notch add more ingredients. My secrets are to never add jealousy, hatred, envy, fear, or for anyone to buy my love. It is either love or not! It is that simple! I can always tell in the beginning. In the beginning, before you make your recipe add discipline, discernment, and detachment. Think logically about the degree of heat you want to bake for your own recipe. As a result, provides a healthy, long, lasting recipe of a relationship. You have the right to turn up or down the level of heat needed! Am I getting a giggle out of you? Well, I must say if the heat is not there, then forget about it. Hey, sometimes you must throw it all away in the trash. Then, start all over again. Remember in the beginning, apply discipline, discernment, and detachment in your recipes always. Then, you never have to bake ever again. Yes, it is that simple my friend.

To recap, a healthy recipe for long lasting relationship you must mix all the right ingredients TOGETHER. Then, your baking experience is heavenly. If you get stuck about what ingredients to add, then take a bath in hot steamy water, lavender oil, and soak in Epson salt. The minerals in Epson salt will drain out all bad elements so your mind is clear of everything. This enables a clear mind for an explosive, yet successful, healthy recipe for life. It does work. Sometimes, if you find yourself scattered it is weight of the world that places pressure on our entire body affecting every organ. Then, your recipe for baking the right relationship becomes jaded. To add, you must mix in sleep. As far as sleep, I must confess I love my sleep. That means so much to me. My secret to sleep is listen to your body, when you feel tired and need rest. People do not really care about your sleep. They all constantly want your time. Remember, you need your energy for successful relationships both professionally and personally. Rest to be your best.

You want forever correct? In order to love others, these special ingredients respect and friendship are the most important ones. Then, love rises really high. Know yourself at first. Ask someone you trust what ingredient your missing. Make adjustments to your own ingredients and start mixing your own recipe. Then, go forward and get that ingredient you have missing called love. As a result, you can appreciate your family, occupation, people in the community, and balance occurs naturally in your life. You will realize what is like to have a healthy, long, lasting recipe for life. At the moment you feel compelled to say what you want for your life recipe, all of the ingredients will come naturally to your mind. What is so crazy, scary and yet so profound are what ingredients we share with each other. We can never take back what was expressed. However, the most challenging ingredient is forgiveness. Forgiveness restores our soul. I know from experience it changes everything. Most people are just too proud to execute this challenging ingredient. After this ingredient called forgiveness is added go get in a mineral, and Epson salt bath. The Epson salt will eliminate all the bad ingredients we carry from others throughout the day. You cannot even imagine what walks into to your life when you walk into a conference room or a home filled with poison. Go check out what Epson salt is made of so you comprehend what occurs to the process of hot, steamy water. I absolutely love it! Do you hear me? Am I coming through to you? Sit on the marble floor or a wooden floor with your feet in front of you. Dump everything on the floor. You must know that crystals, marble, minerals, rid yourself of bad energy and enable good energy to settle inwardly. Just ask me. I will explain. One of darling clients, a fitness expert taught me this in McKinney, Texas as her talent agent and her friend. Remember, we are filled with energy from cell phones, computers, and microwaves throughout the day. Go do the Epson salt and mineral bath as soon as possible. I promise you will see how invigorating your body and mind are afterwards.

Consequently, this leads to some ingredient concerns in life. Go ahead to chapter three and list some ingredients missing in your own life recipe. I can list so many. Then, execute a plan to eliminate each ingredient by process of elimination. Add new ingredients to replace the old ingredients that caused your recipe to fail.

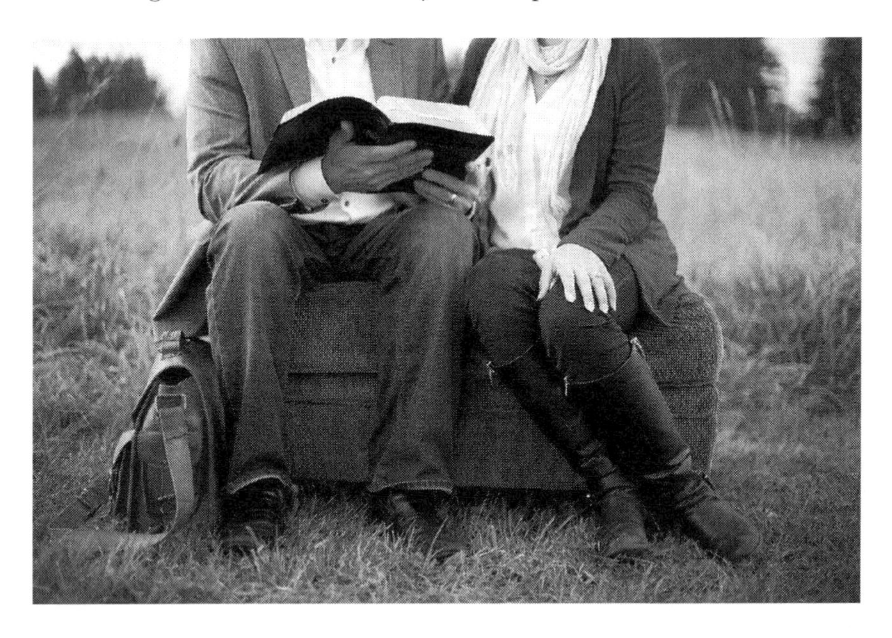

Quote: It is easy to say "I love you"! It is the response we are afraid of.

Ask for strength from our heavenly father! Then, give him your entire recipe and trust he will bake it at the perfect temperature.

Chapter 3

INGREDIENT CONCERNS

Ingredient concern
Answered ingredient concern (Circle: Yes or No)

Ingredient concerns

Date:

Ingredient Answered: Yes or No (circle it)

Ingredient concerns

Date:

Ingredient Answered: Yes or No (circle it)

Ingredient concerns

Date:

Ingredient Answered: Yes or No (circle it)

Ingredient concerns

Date:

Ingredient Answered: Yes or No (circle it)

Ingredient concerns

Date:

____
____
____
____

Ingredient Answered: Yes or No (circle it)

Ingredient concerns

Date:

____
____
____
____

Ingredient Answered: Yes or No (circle it)

Ingredient concerns

Date:

____
____
____
____

Ingredient Answered: Yes or No (circle it)

Ingredient concerns

Date:

____
____
____
____

Ingredient Answered: Yes or No (circle it)

Ingredient concerns

Date:

Ingredient Answered: Yes or No (circle it)

Ingredient concerns

Date:

Ingredient Answered: Yes or No (circle it)

Ingredient concerns

Date:

Ingredient Answered: Yes or No (circle it)

Ingredient concerns

Date:

Ingredient Answered: Yes or No (circle it)

Ingredient concerns

Date:

____

____

____

____

Ingredient Answered: Yes or No (circle it)

Quote: Don't let your aim ever stray. You may never get that stray back.

THE END.

Donations/Contact

Wolf Entertainment productions and the CHD Community appreciate your generosity. We make it easy to donate.

If you go to http://silentcriesmovie.com you will find the donate page on the site simply click on it and all donations go thru pay pal which is then handled thru our fiscal sponsor Carol Dean at From the heart productions. This is how everyone who donates is assured a tax deduction for their contribution. You can also find Carol Dean›s website link on the http://silentcriesmovie.com site as well. If you have Any questions or problems please contact me. Again, on behalf of the entire CHD and the Silent Cries Team we thank you very much.

Wolf Entertainment Productions: Phillip Wolf 1-866-788-8869

For any more information concerning this book contact Ms. Mollie Ann Holt at 310-321-2390 or mollieannholt@gmail.com.

I.S.B.N.
$1.00 goes to the charity called, Silent Cries
Film project concerning C.H.D. congestive, heart, disease.

Made in United States
Orlando, FL
25 March 2022